FOOD NOT FOOD

A VISUAL JOURNEY OF REAL FOODS
AND THEIR LOOK-ALIKES

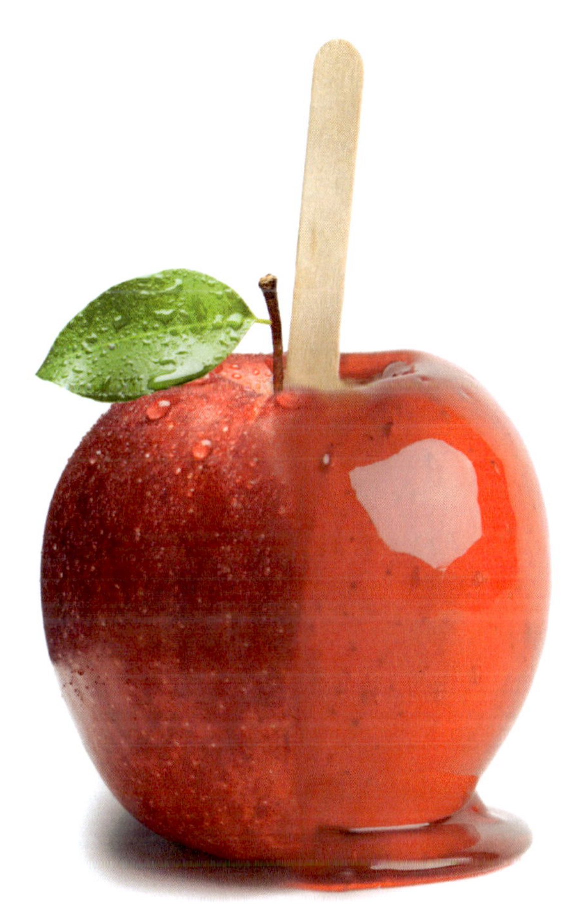

by

ALLISON BERGMAN and MARCELLE SIRKUS

Sweet Pepper Publishing
California, U.S.A.

INTRODUCTION

On the following pages we share awe-inspiring pictures of natural foods alongside products that look like food, sometimes designed so cleverly to fool the eye, we don't even question it — until we read the ingredients!

Food is defined as a substance consisting essentially of protein, carbohydrates, fat and other nutrients used to sustain growth and vital processes, and to provide energy. However, many of the additives and preservatives we consume don't meet that definition.

For the record, we are neither professional nutritionists nor members of any regulatory agency. But in our opinion, not everything considered edible should be called food.

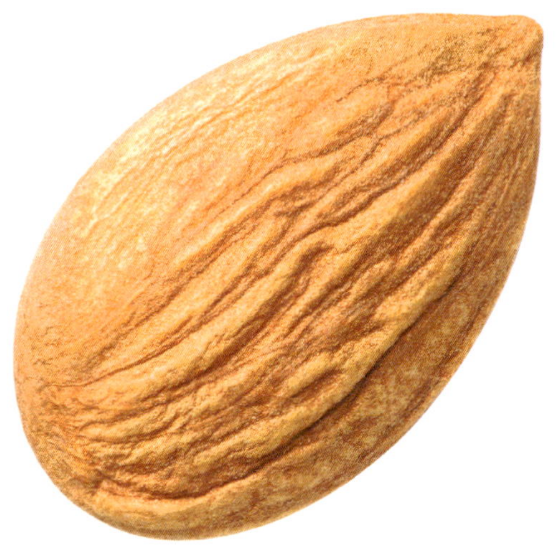

Almond.

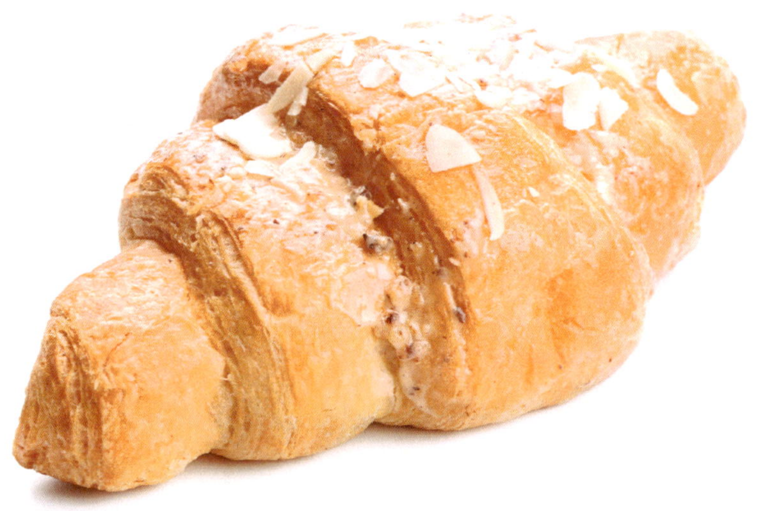

Wheat Flour, Malted Barley Flour, Niacin, Reduced Iron, Thiamine Mononitrate, Riboflavin, Folic Acid, Cream, Water, Milk, Sugar, Eggs, Yeast, Salt, Ascorbic Acid, Enzymes, Soybean and Palm Oil, Propylene Glycol Monoesters, Mono- and Diglycerides, Soy Lecithin, BHT, Citric Acid, Dextrose, Modified Corn Starch, Sodium Aluminum Phosphate, Sodium Bicarbonate, Soy Protein, Polysorbate 60, Natural and Artificial Flavors, Gum Arabic, Corn Syrup Solids, Tetrasodium Pyrophosphate, Sodium Propionate, Calcium Acetate, Guar Gum, Potassium Sorbate, Xanthan Gum, High Fructose Corn Syrup, Benzoic Acid, Cellulose Gel and Gum, Yellow #5 and #6, Magnesium Stearate, Almonds, Pectin, Carrageenan, Sodium Citrate, Sodium Metabisulfite, Sodium Phosphate, and Paprika.

FOOD

NOT FOOD

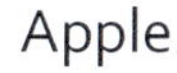

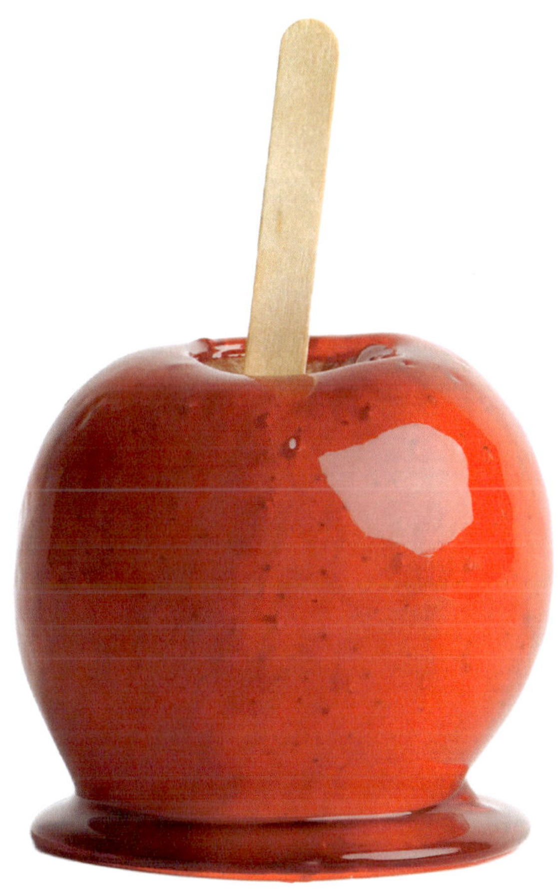

Apple.

Apple, Sugar, Dextrose, Red #40, and Artificial Flavors.

FOOD

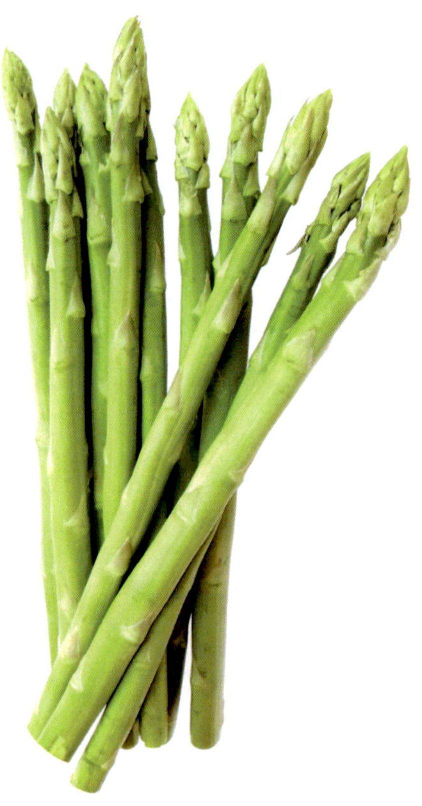

Asparagus.

NOT FOOD

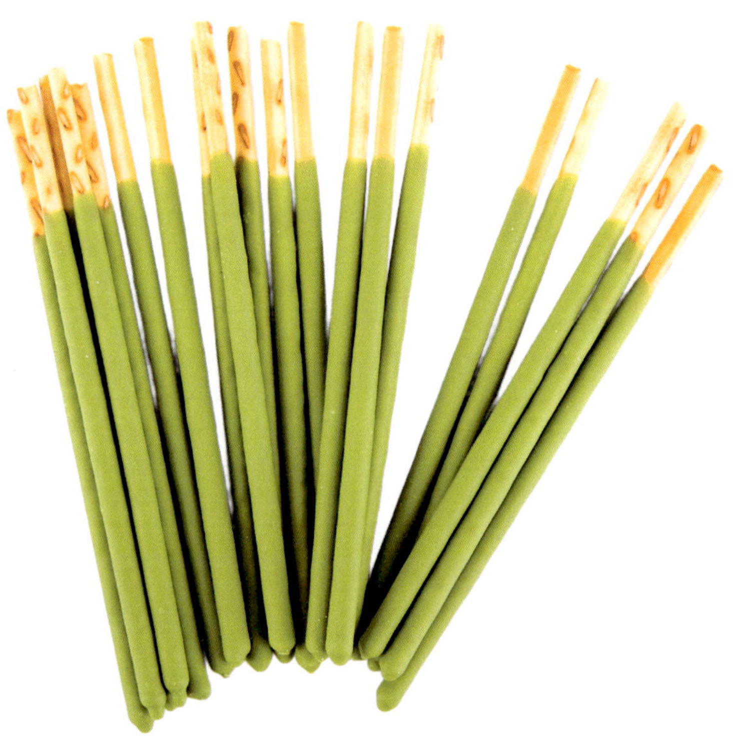

Wheat Flour, Ferrous Fumarate, Niacinamide, Thiamin Mononitrate, Riboflavin, Folic Acid, Sugar, Fully Hydrogenated Palm Oil, Whole Milk Powder, Lactose, Modified Food Starch, Inulin, Palm Oil, Malt Extract, Green Tea Powder, Artificial Flavor, Soy Lecithin, Salt, Sodium Bicarbonate, and Saccharomyces Cerevisiae.

FOOD

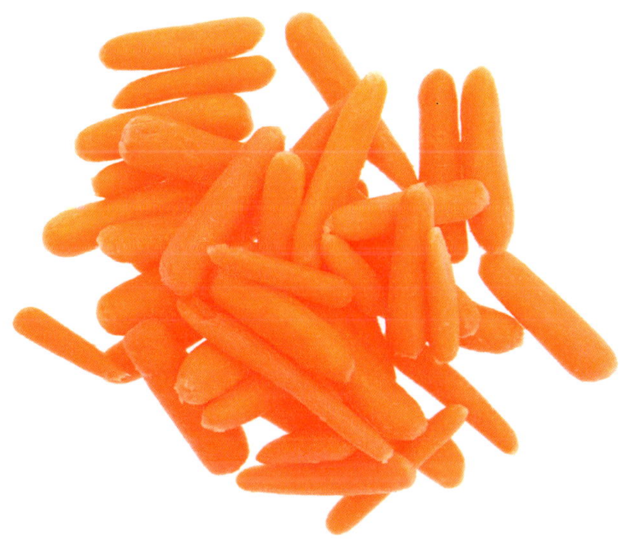

Baby-cut Carrots.

NOT FOOD

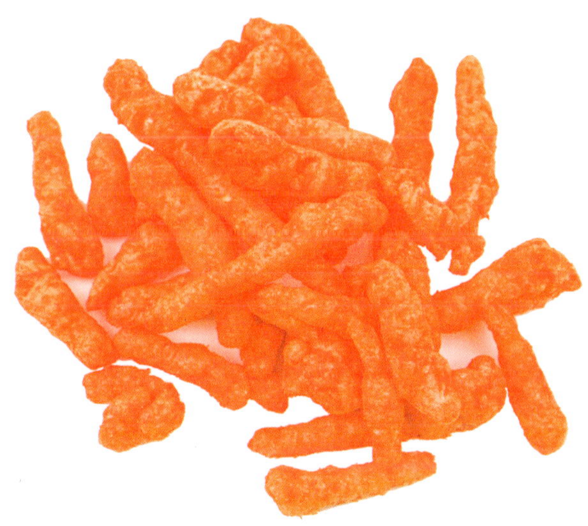

Corn Meal, Ferrous Sulfate, Niacin, Thiamin Mononitrate, Riboflavin, Folic Acid, Corn, Canola and/or Sunflower Oil, Cheese Seasoning, Whey, Milk, Cheese Cultures, Salt, Enzymes, Maltodextrin, Natural and Artificial Flavors, Whey Protein Concentrate, Monosodium Glutamate, Lactic Acid, Citric Acid, and Yellow #6.

FOOD

NOT FOOD

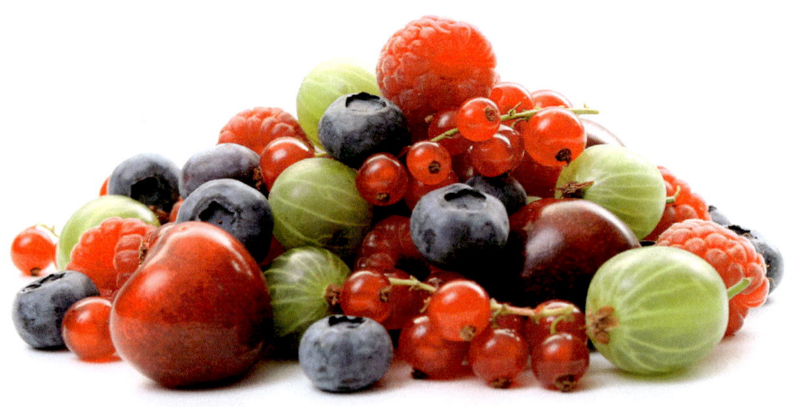

Berries.

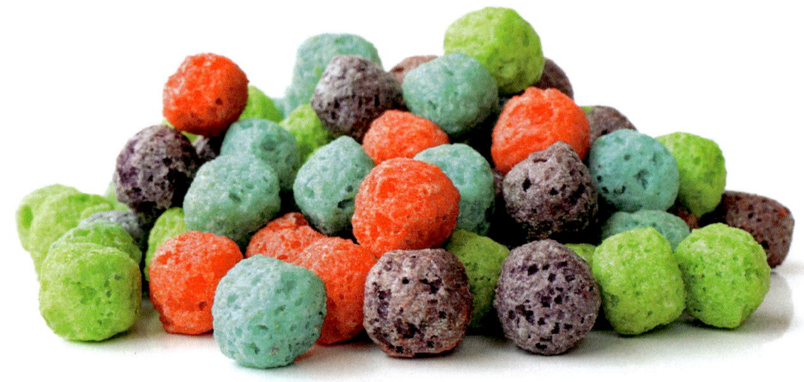

Corn Flour, Sugar, Oat Flour, Brown Sugar, Palm and/or Coconut Oil, Salt, Sodium Citrate, Natural and Artificial Flavor, Malic Acid, Red #40, Blue #1, Reduced Iron, Yellow #5, Niacinamide, Thiamin Mononitrate, BHT, Pyridoxine Hydrochloride, Riboflavin, and Folic Acid.

FOOD

NOT FOOD

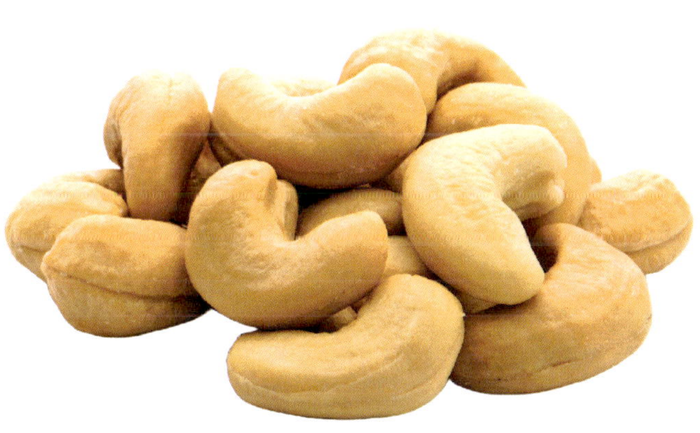

Cashews.

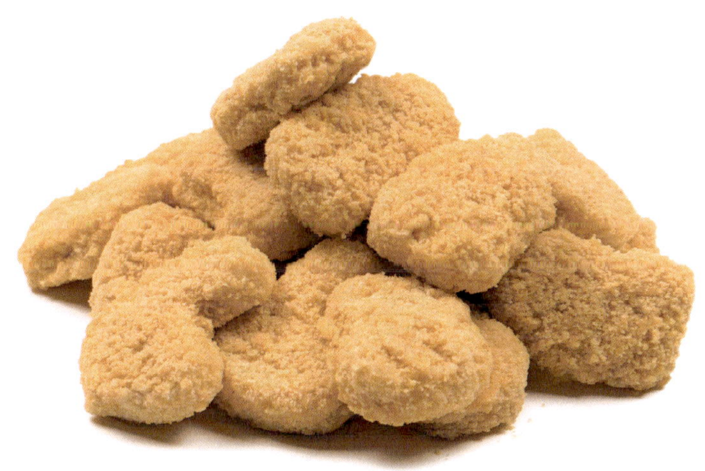

Chicken Meat, Water, Bleached Wheat Flour, Salt, Dextrose, Yeast, Soybean Oil, Spices, Extractives of Paprika, Textured Soy Flour, Yellow Corn Flour, Corn Starch, Sugar, Autolyzed Yeast Extract, Modified Corn Starch, Garlic Powder, Guar Gum, Sodium Bicarbonate, Monocalcium Phosphate, Sodium Tripolyphosphate, and Flavorings.

FOOD

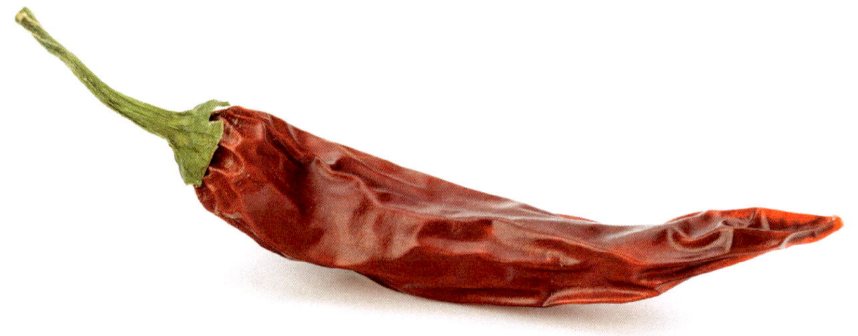

Cayenne Pepper.

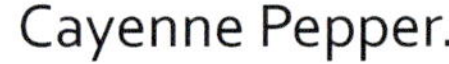

NOT FOOD

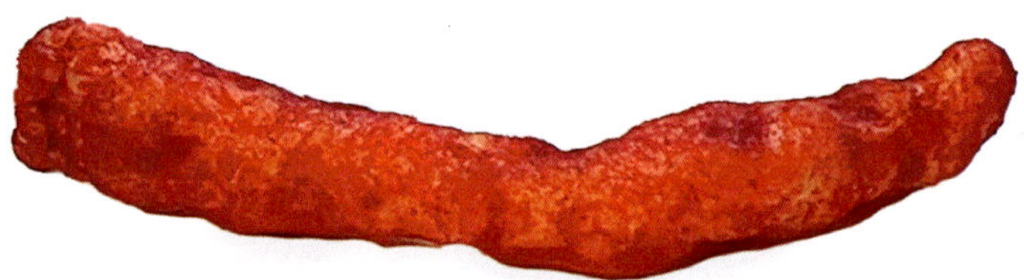

Corn Meal, Ferrous Sulfate, Niacin, Thiamin Mononitrate, Riboflavin, Folic Acid, Vegetable Oil, Salt, Maltodextrin, Yeast Extract, Monosodium Glutamate, Potassium Salt, Citric Acid, Sugar, Artificial Color, Red #40 Lake, Yellow #6 Lake, Yellow #6, Yellow #5, Milk, Cheese Cultures, Enzymes, Onion Powder, Whey, Whey Protein Concentrate, Garlic Powder, Natural Flavors, Buttermilk, Sodium Diacetate, Disodium Inosinate, and Disodium.

FOOD

NOT FOOD

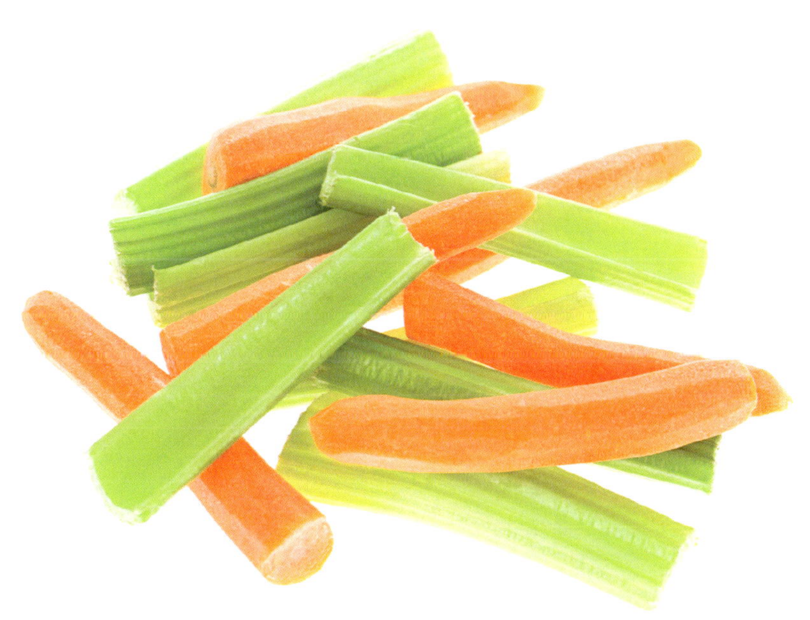

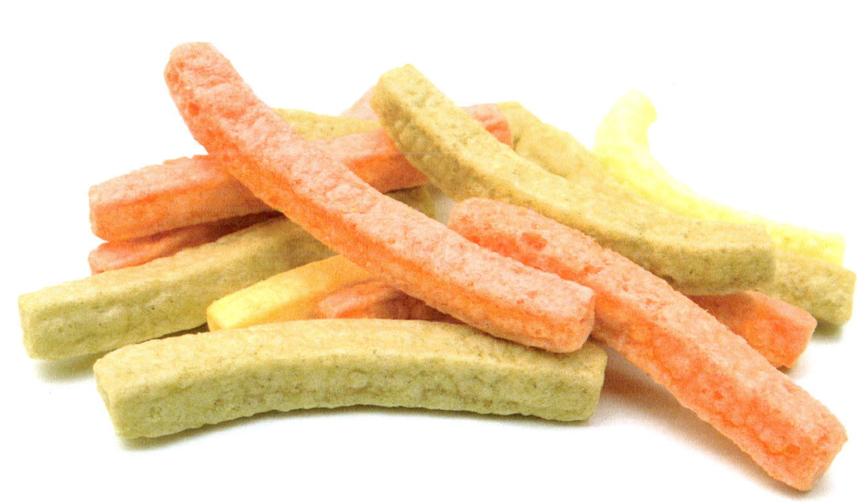

Celery and Carrots.

Potato Starch, Potato Flour, Dehydrated Spinach, Tomato Paste, Salt, Cane Sugar, Corn Starch, Potassium Chloride, Turmeric, Beetroot Powder, Canola Oil and/or Safflower Oil and/or Sunflower Oil, Natural Flavors, Coconut Oil, Corn Maltodextrin, Spices, Yeast Extract, Milk Ingredients, Cultures, Dextrose, Dehydrated Tomato, Citric Acid, Cultured Skim Milk, Sugar, Lactic Acid, Malic Acid, Vinegar, and Sodium Caseinate.

FOOD

NOT FOOD

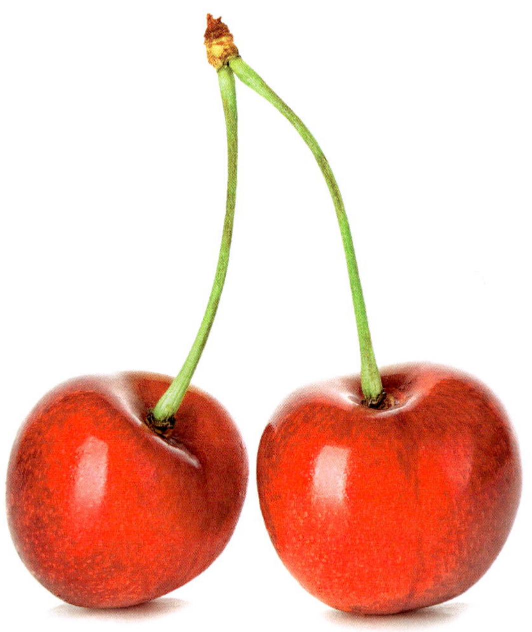

Cherries.

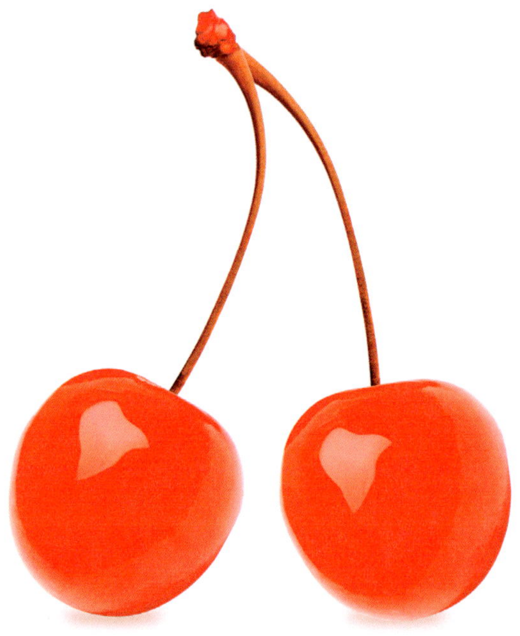

Cherries, Water, Corn Syrup, High Fructose Corn Syrup, Malic Acid, Citric Acid, Natural and Artificial Flavor, Potassium Sorbate, Sodium Benzoate, FD&C Red #40, and Sulfur Dioxide.

FOOD

NOT FOOD

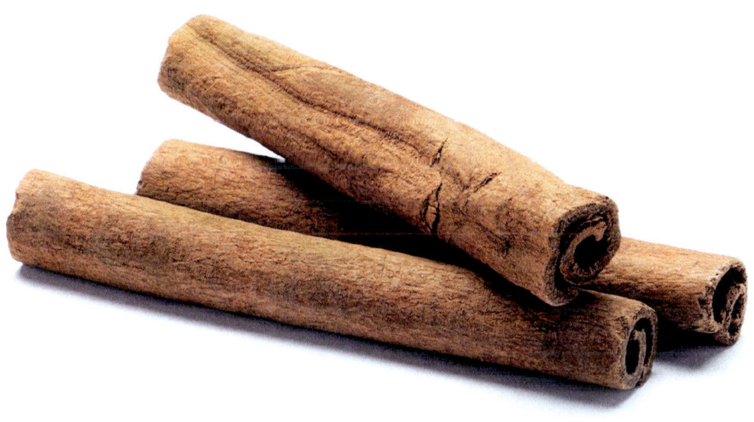

Cinnamon Sticks.

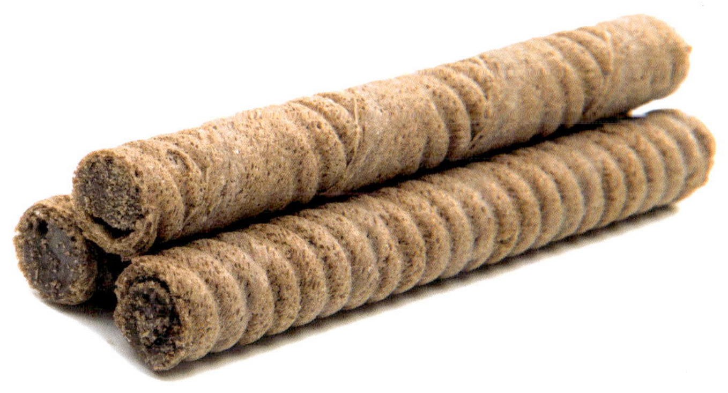

Sugar, Wheat Flour, Palm Oil, Maltodextrin, Dextrose, Cocoa Processed with Alkali, Hazelnuts, Whey, Rice Flour, Soy Lecithin, Caramel Color, Milk, Salt, Mono- and Diglycerides, Enzymes, Ascorbyl Palmitate, Alpha Tocopherol, Reduced Iron, Zinc Oxide, Riboflavin, Thiamine Mononitrate, and Folic Acid.

FOOD

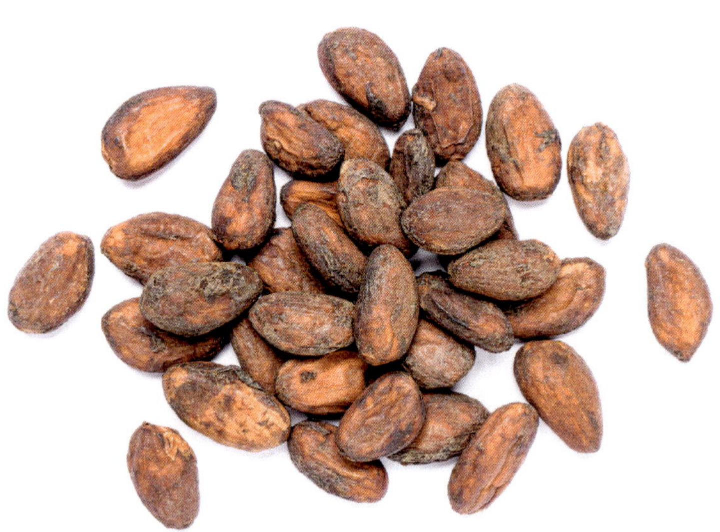

Cocoa Beans.

NOT FOOD

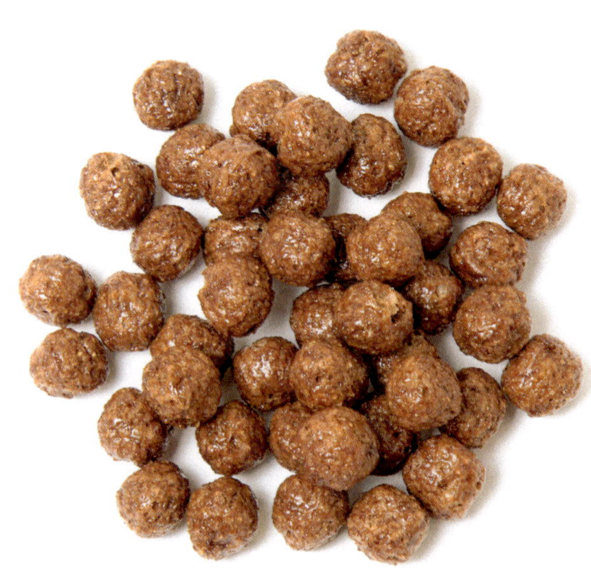

Whole Grain Corn, Sugar, Rice Flour, Corn Syrup, Cocoa Processed with Alkali, Canola and/or Sunflower Oil, Salt, Caramel Color, Annatto Extract, Baking Soda, Natural Flavor, Tricalcium Phosphate, Calcium Carbonate, Sodium Ascorbate, Mineral Nutrients, Niacinamide, Pyridoxine Hydrochloride, Thiamin Mononitrate, Palmitate, Riboflavin, Folic Acid, Vitamin B12, and Vitamin D3.

FOOD

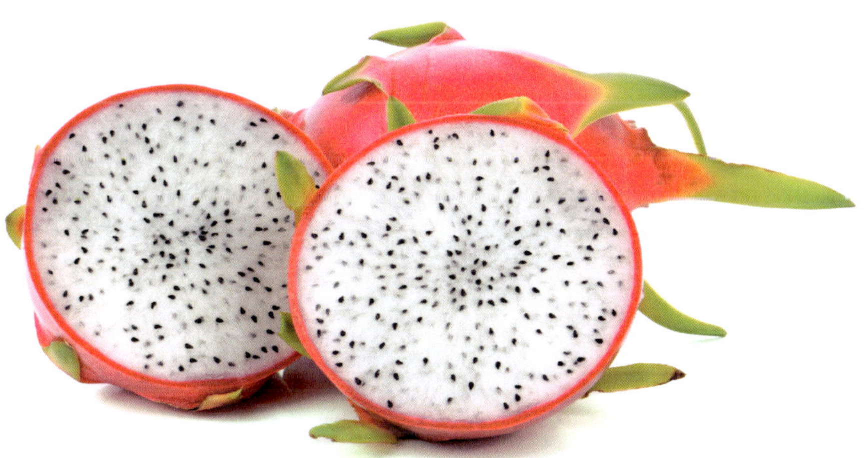

Dragon Fruit.

NOT FOOD

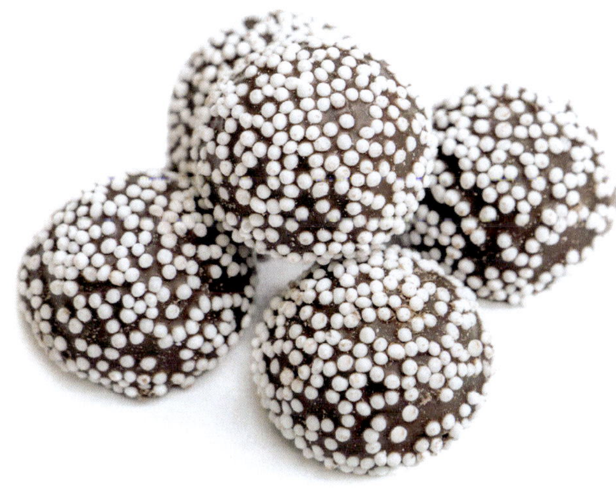

Sugar, Chocolate, Milkfat, Cocoa Butter, Soy Lecithin, Natural Flavor, Corn Starch, Carnauba Wax, and Lac Resin.

FOOD

NOT FOOD

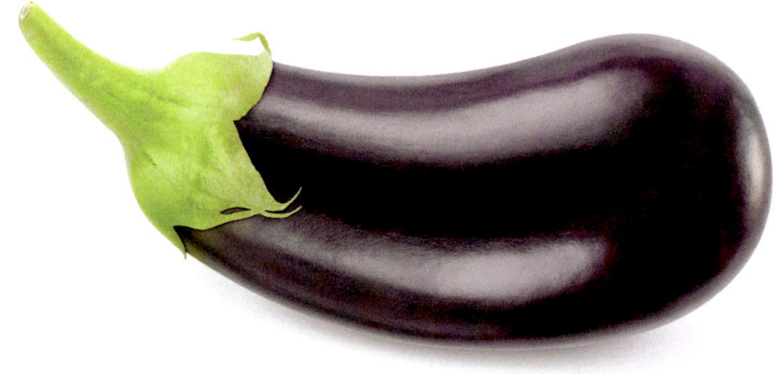

Eggplant.

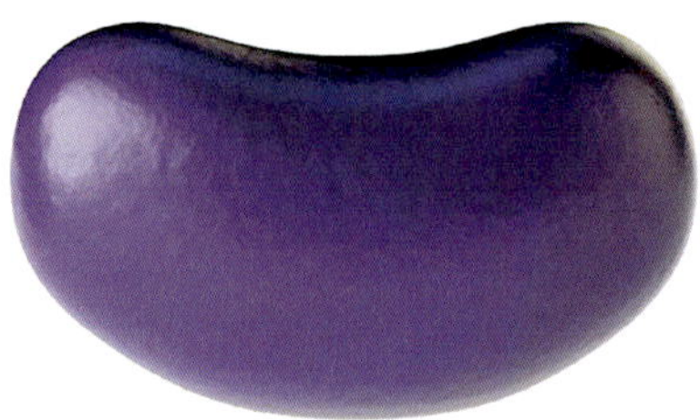

Sugar, Corn Syrup, Modified Food Starch, Citric Acid, Sodium Lactate, Tartaric Acid, Grape Juice Concentrate, Acacia Gum, Natural and Artificial Flavor, Color Added, Red #40, Blue #1, Beeswax, Carnauba Wax, and Confectioner's Glaze.

FOOD

NOT FOOD

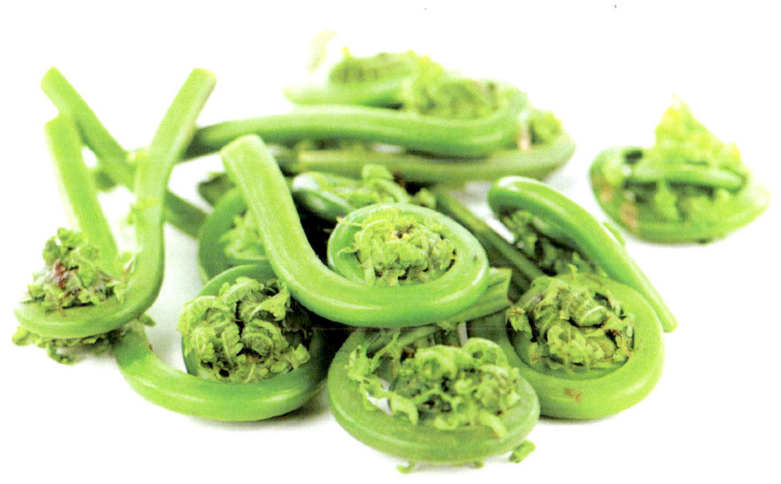

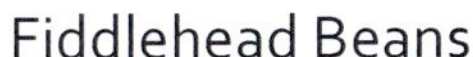

Fiddlehead Beans.

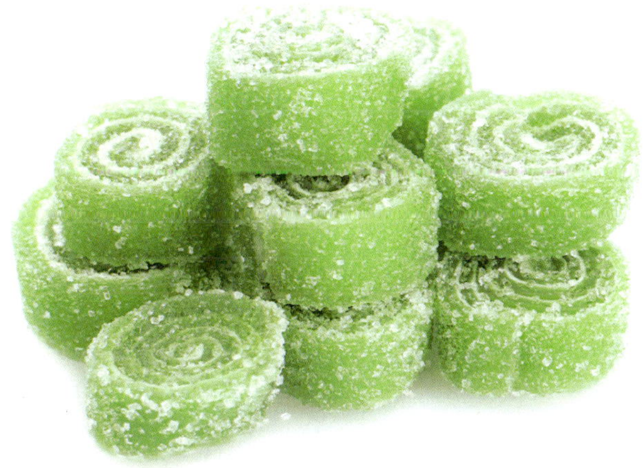

Sugar, Corn Starch, Water, Desiccated Coconut,
Citric Acid, Apple Flavor, and Coloring Agent.

FOOD

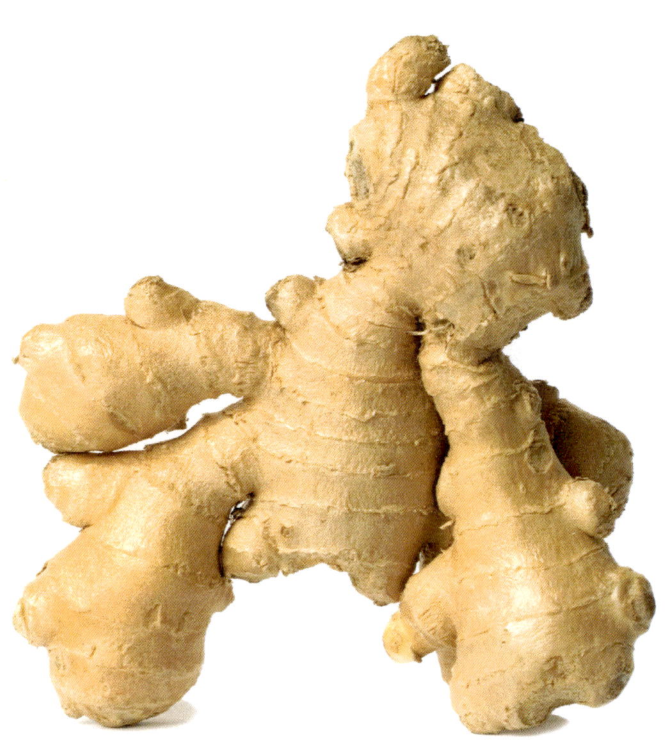

Ginger Root.

NOT FOOD

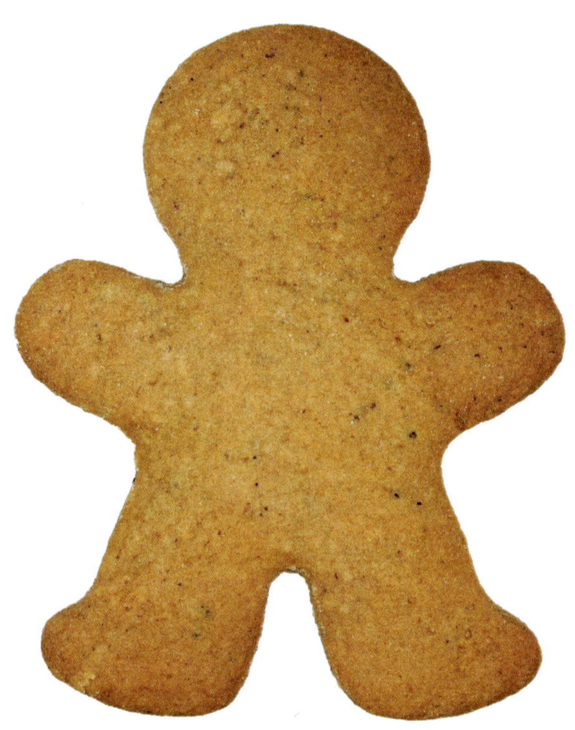

Wheat Flour, Niacin, Reduced Iron, Ascorbic Acid, Thiamine Mononitrate, Riboflavin, Enzyme, Sugar, Canola Oil, Palm Oil, Invert Sugar, Water, Spices, Caramel Color, Salt, Baking Soda, Eggs, Soy Lecithin, Nonfat Dry Milk, Soy and Sugar from Genetically Modified Crops, and Bioengineered Food Ingredients.

FOOD

NOT FOOD

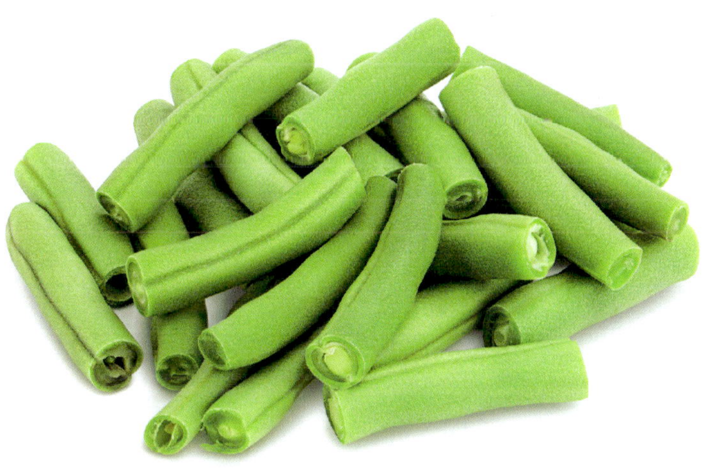

Green Beans.

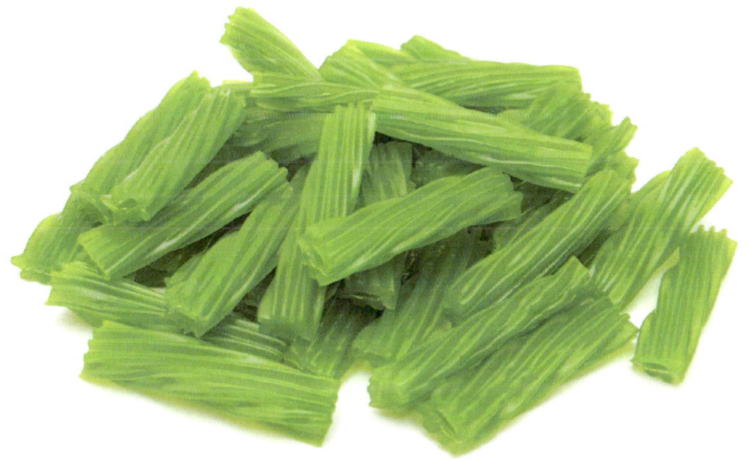

Wheat, Iron, Niacin, Thiamin, Riboflavin, Folic Acid, Corn Syrup, High Fructose Corn Syrup, Sugar, Water, Modified Food Starch, Artificial Flavor, Apple Juice Concentrate, Citric Acid, Salt, Malic Acid, Palm Oil, Soy Lecithin, Glycerin, Soy Mono- and Diglycerides, Ascorbic Acid, FD&C Yellow #5, FD&C Yellow #5 Lake, and FD&C Blue #1 Lake.

FOOD

NOT FOOD

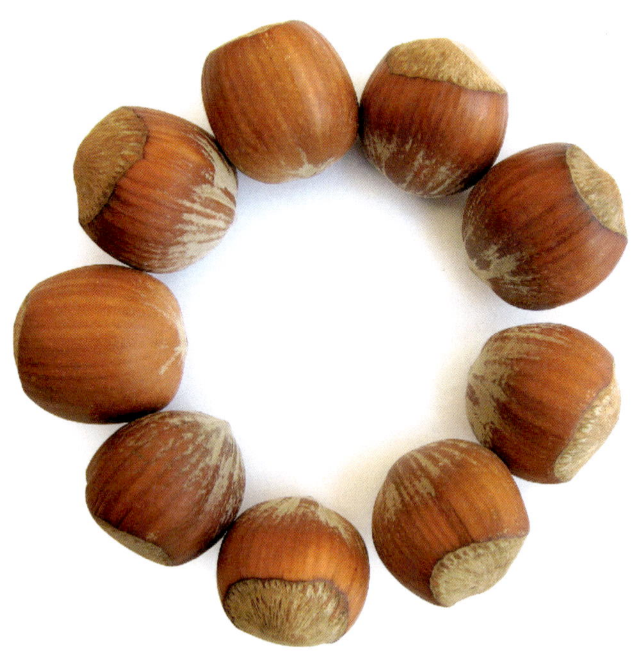

Hazelnuts.

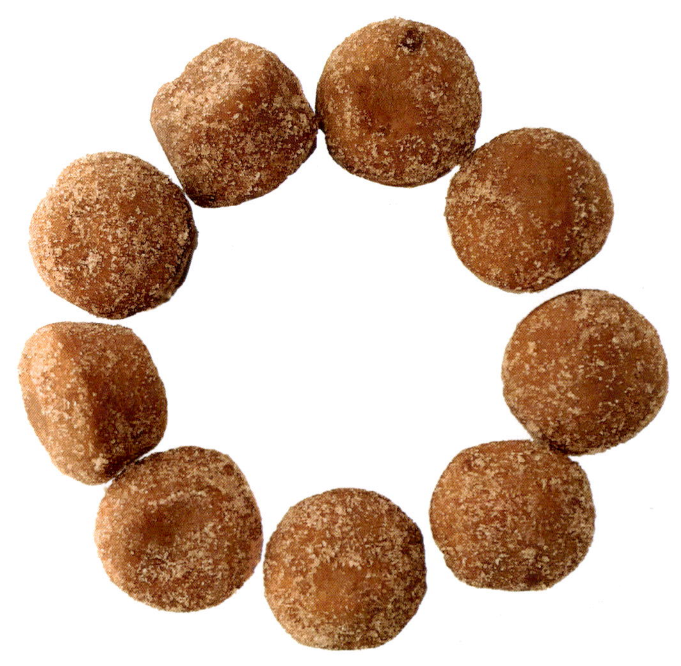

Wheat Flour, Niacin, Reduced Iron, Thiamine Mononitrate, Riboflavin, Folic Acid, Sugar, Water, Palm Oil, Dextrose, Soybean Oil, Defatted Soy Flour, Whey, Sodium Acid Pyrophosphate, Baking Soda, Egg Yolk with Sodium Silicoaluminate, Salt, Wheat Starch, Milk Protein Concentrate, Mono- and Diglycerides, Natural and Artificial Flavor, Gum Arabic, Enzymes, Beta Carotene, Calcium Carbonate, Calcium Sulfate, Agar, Locust Bean Gum, and Sodium Phosphate.

FOOD

NOT FOOD

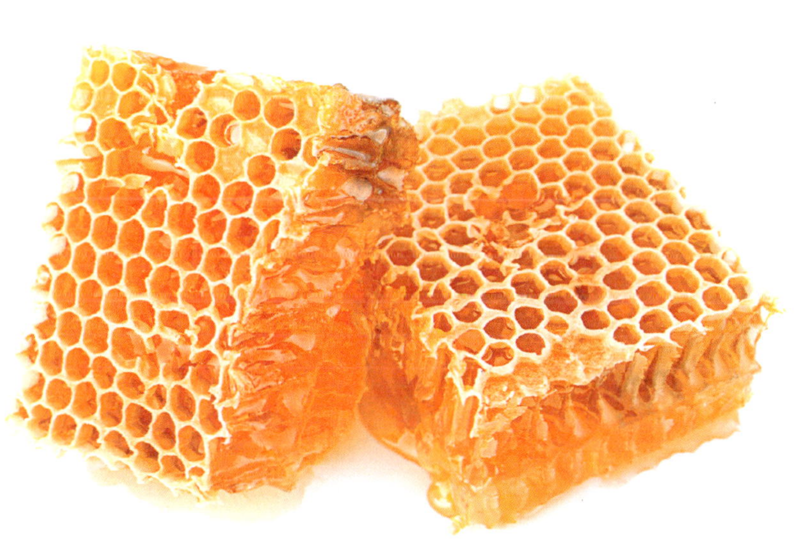

Honeycomb.

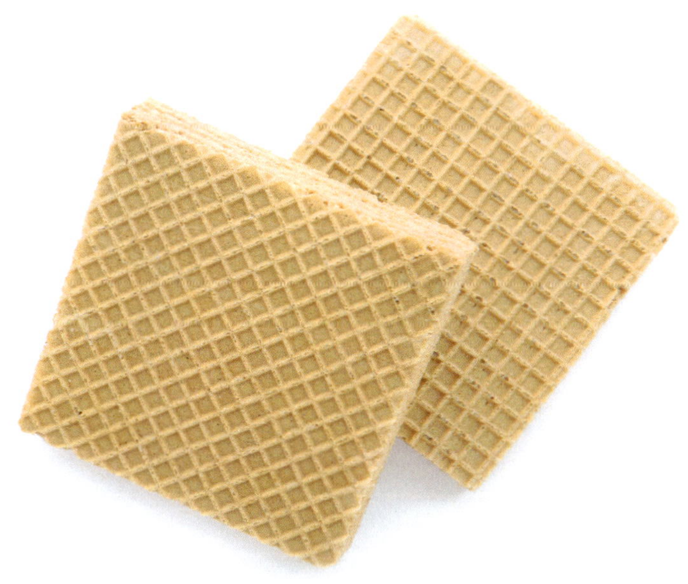

Sugar, Wheat Flour, Malted Barley Flour, Niacin, Reduced Iron, Thiamin Mononitrate, Riboflavin, Folic Acid, Palm Oil, Dextrose, Canola Oil, Artificial Flavor, Soy Lecithin, Salt, Baking Soda, Yellow #5, Yellow #6, Red #3, and Citric Acid.

FOOD

NOT FOOD

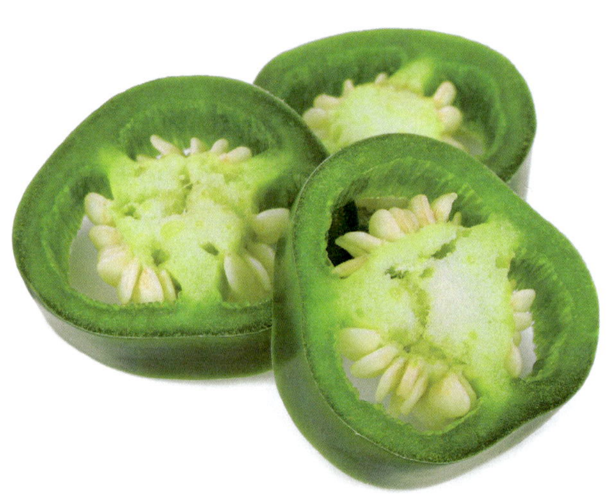

Jalapeño.

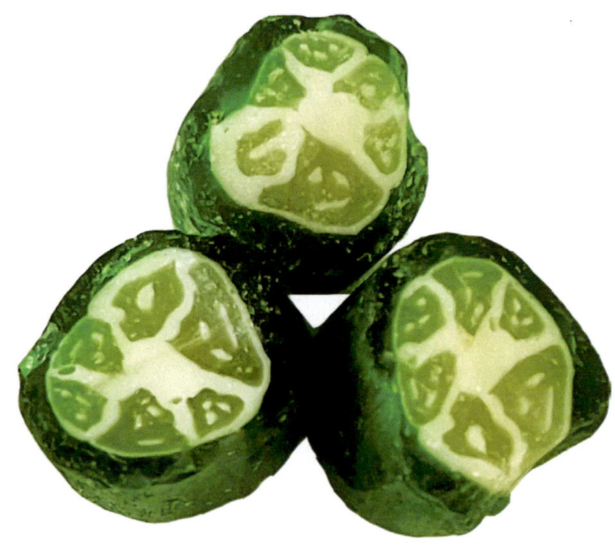

Sugar, Corn Syrup, Citric Acid, Artificial and Natural Flavors, Titanium Dioxide Color, Yellow #5, Red #40, Blue #1, Red #3, Yellow #6, and Soy Lecithin.

FOOD

NOT FOOD

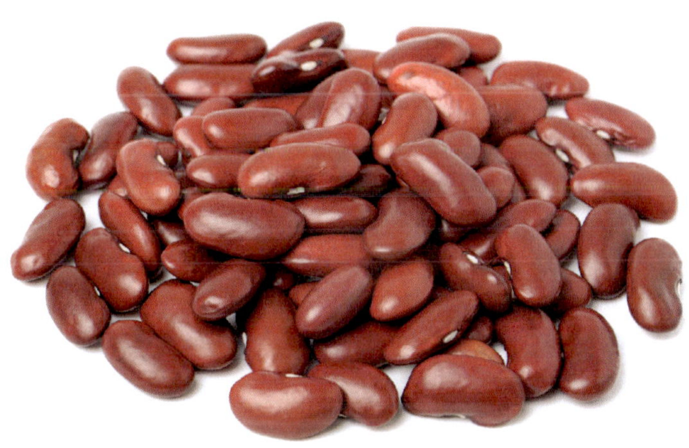

Kidney Beans.

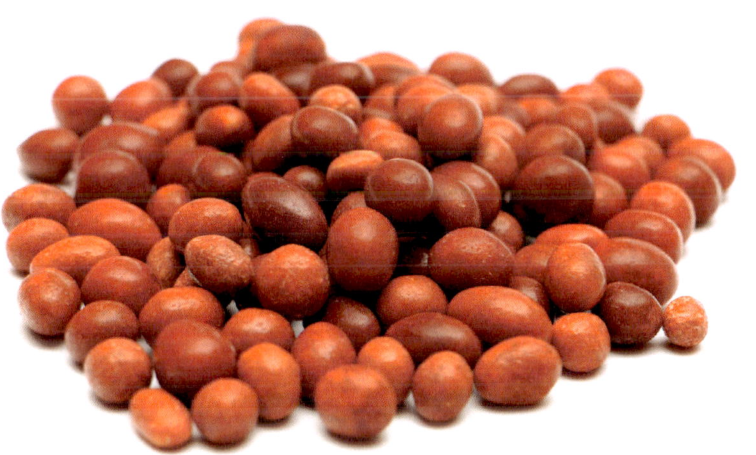

Sugar, Peanuts, Corn Syrup, Modified Food Starch, Acacia, Shellac, Artificial Flavor, Carnauba Wax, White Mineral Oil, Red #40, Yellow #5, Yellow #6, Blue #2, Tree Nuts and their Derivatives, Corn and its Derivatives, and Peanuts and their Derivatives.

FOOD

NOT FOOD

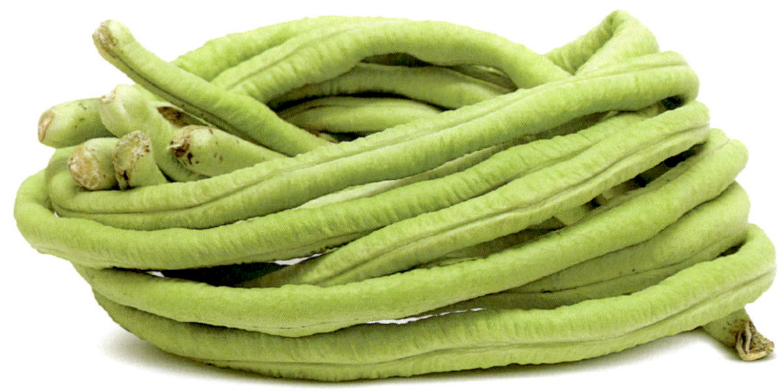

Long Beans.

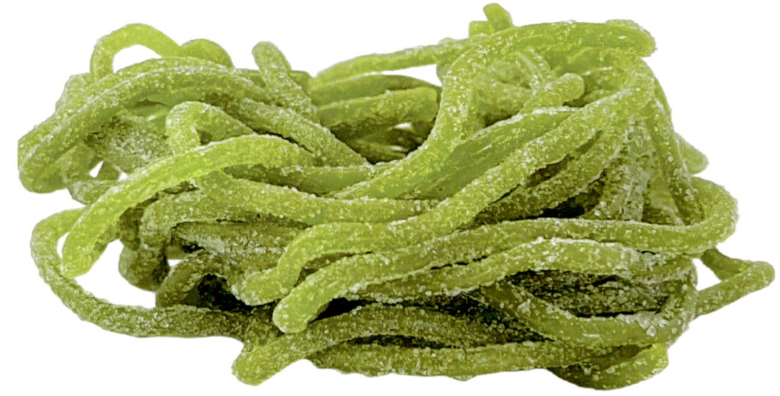

Sugar, Glucose Syrup, Wheat Flour, Malic Acid, Palm Fat, Citric Acid, Apple Juice Concentrate, Sorbitol, Corn Starch, Mono- and Diglycerides of Fatty Acids, Flavoring, and Copper Complexes of Chlorophyllins.

FOOD

NOT FOOD

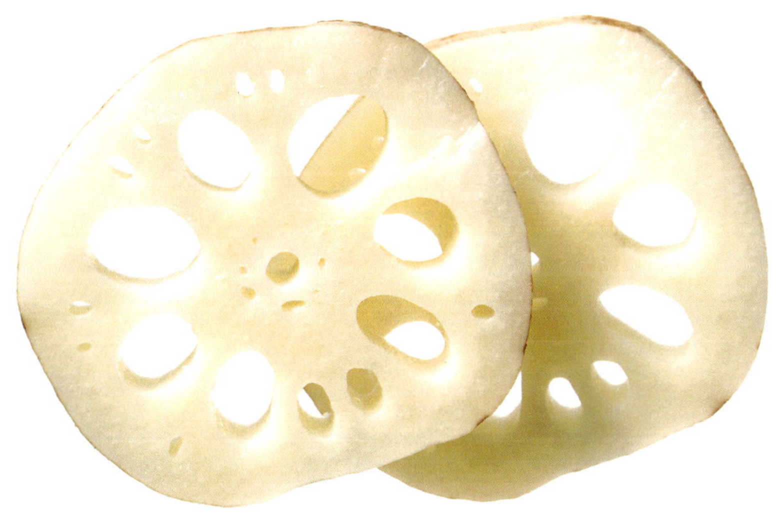

Lotus Root.

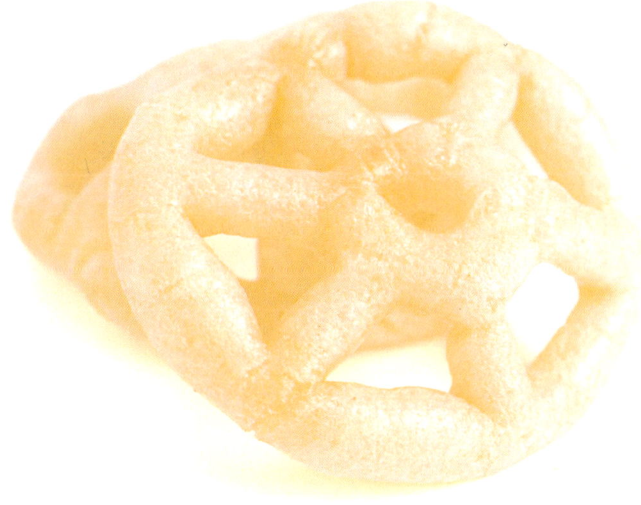

Sugar, Wheat Starch, Water, Cottonseed Oil, Wheat Flour, Egg, Partially Hydrogenated Palm Oil, Soy Lecithin, Nonfat Milk, Iodized Salt, Baking Soda, Sodium Aluminium Sulfate, Calcium Sulfate, Monocalcıum Phosphate, TBHQ, Thiamin Mononitrate, Riboflavin, Niacin, Folic Acid, Ferrous Sulfate, and Zinc Oxide.

FOOD	NOT FOOD

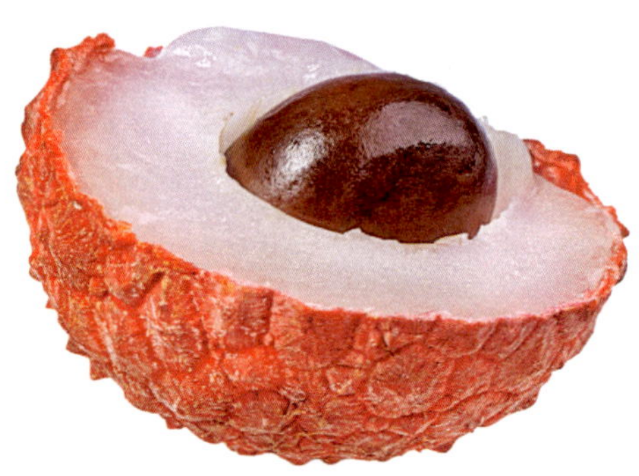

Lychee.

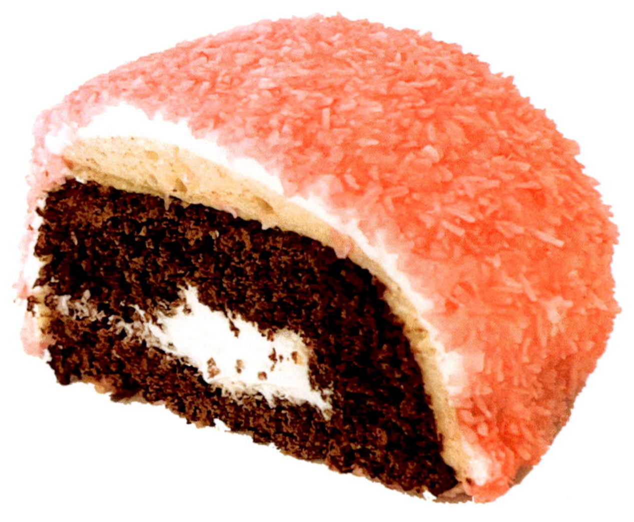

Wheat Flour, Niacin, Reduced Iron, Thiamine Mononitrate, Riboflavin, Folic Acid, Water, High Fructose Corn Syrup, Sugar, Canola, Soybean and/or Cottonseed Oil, Eggs, Cocoa Processed with Alkali, Baking Soda, Sodium Aluminum Phosphate, Monocalcium Phosphate, Salt, Mono- and Diglycerides, Polysorbate 60, Soy Lecithin, Artificial Flavor, Yellow #5, Red #40, and Blue #1.

FOOD

NOT FOOD

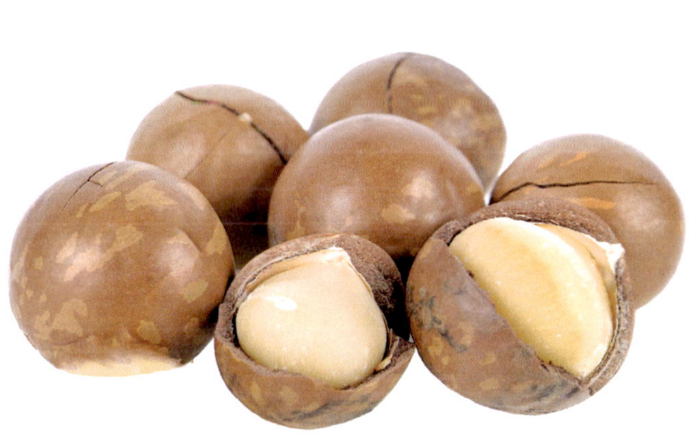

Macadamia Nuts.

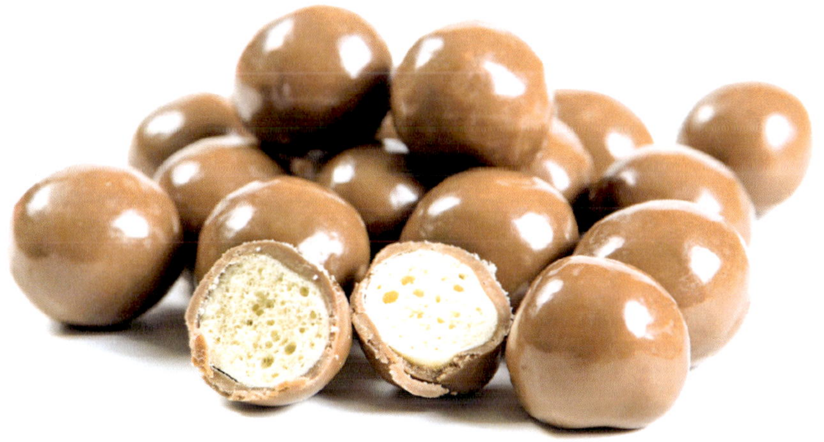

Sugar, Corn Syrup Solids, Whey, Hydrogenated Palm Kernel Oil, Palm Kernel Oil, Corn Syrup, Cocoa, Barley Malt, Wheat Flour, Milk, Salt, Baking Soda, Sorbitan Tristearate, Lecithin, Confectioner's Glaze, Artificial Flavor, Tapioca Dextrin, and Calcium Carbonate.

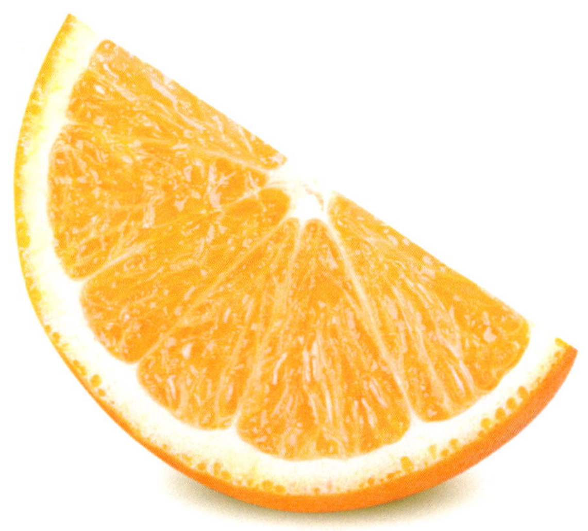

FOOD

Orange.

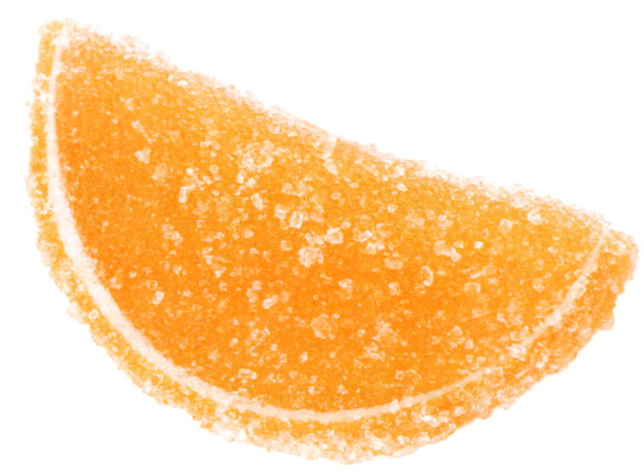

NOT FOOD

Sugar, Corn Syrup, Agar, Citric Acid, Titanium Dioxide, Natural and Artificial Flavors, Red #4, Blue #1, Yellow #5, and Yellow #6.

FOOD

NOT FOOD

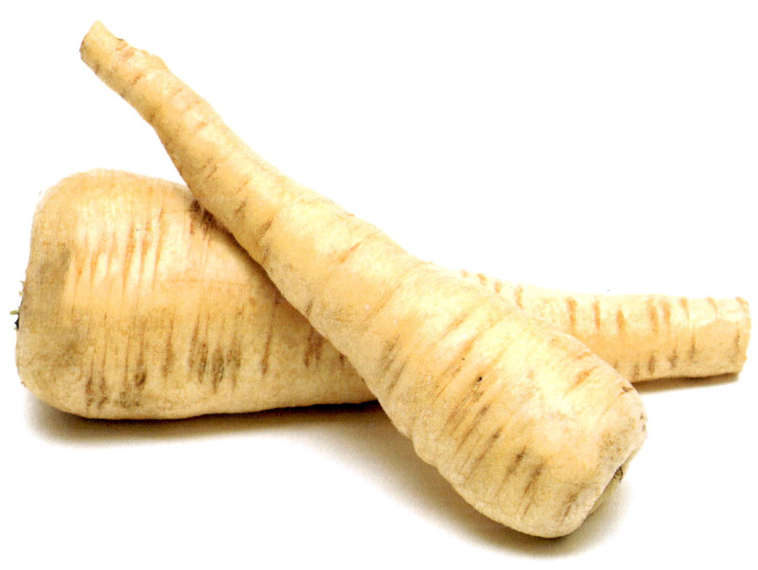

Parsnips.

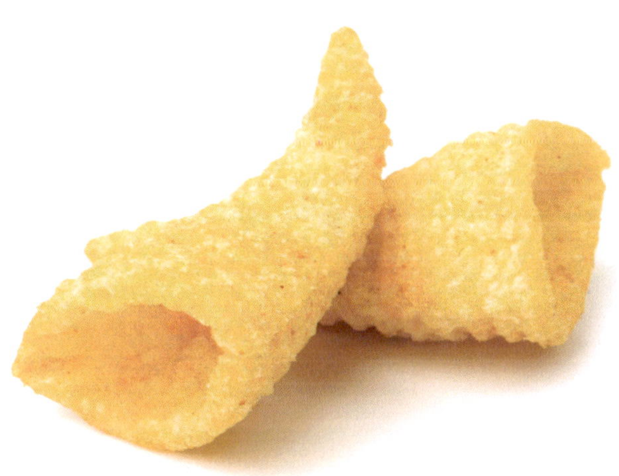

Degermed Yellow Corn Meal, Coconut Oil and/or Palm Kernel Oil, Sugar, Salt, Baking Soda, and BHT.

FOOD

NOT FOOD

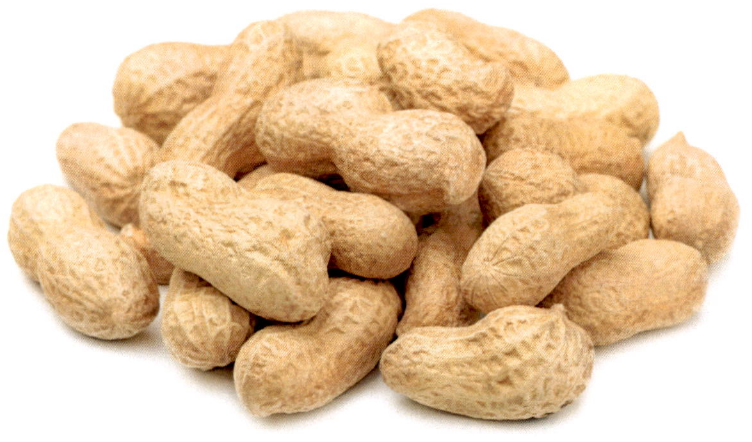

Peanuts.

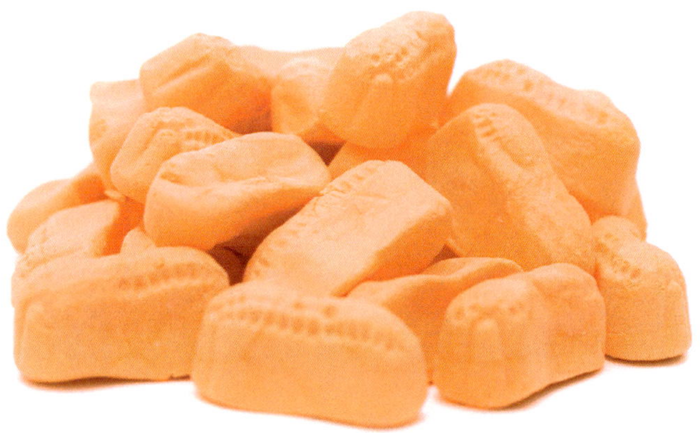

Sugar, Corn Syrup, Gelatin, Pectin, Artificial Flavor, Yellow #6, Yellow #5, and Red #40.

FOOD

NOT FOOD

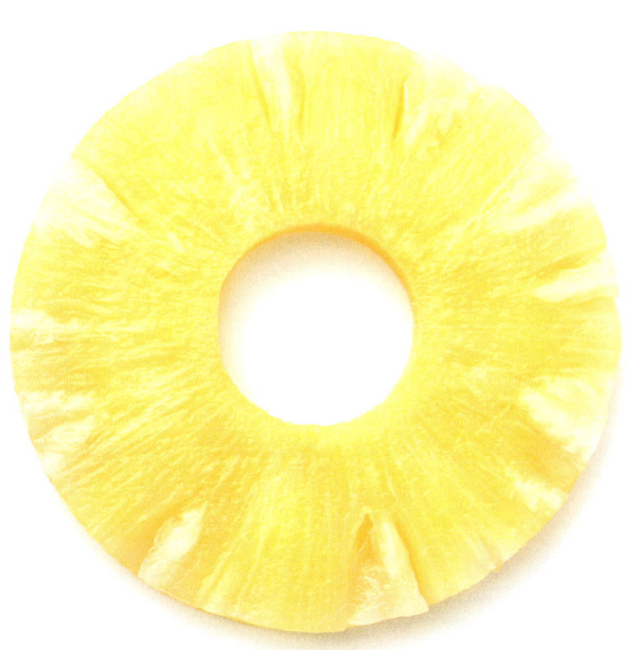

Pineapple.

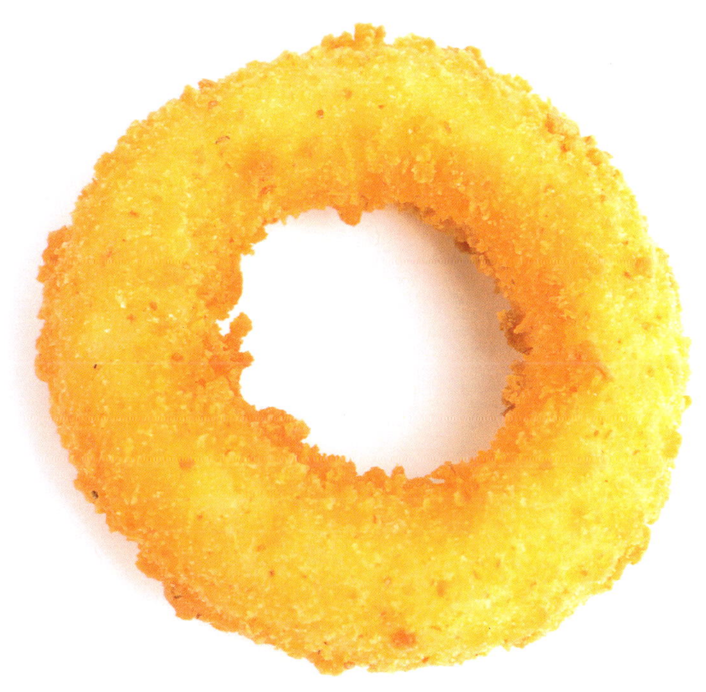

Onions, Bleached Wheat Flour, Water, Soybean and/or Canola Oil, Wheat Flour, Yellow Corn Flour, Dextrose, Expeller Pressed Sunflower Oil, Monocalcium Phosphate, Sodium Bicarbonate, Polysorbate 8o, Salt, and Bioengineered Food Ingredients.

FOOD

NOT FOOD

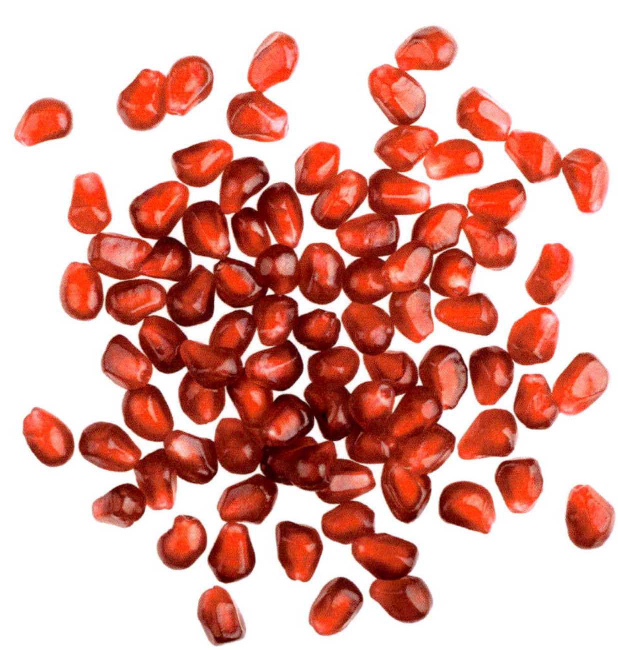

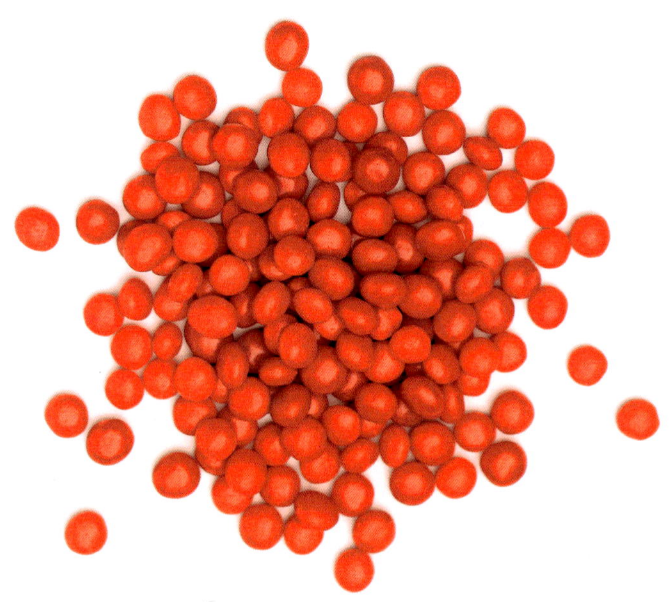

Pomegranate Seeds.

Sugar, Corn Syrup, Gum Arabic, Artificial Flavor, Shellac, Carnauba Wax, White Mineral Oil, Red #40, Cornstarch, and Sunflower Lecithin.

FOOD

NOT FOOD

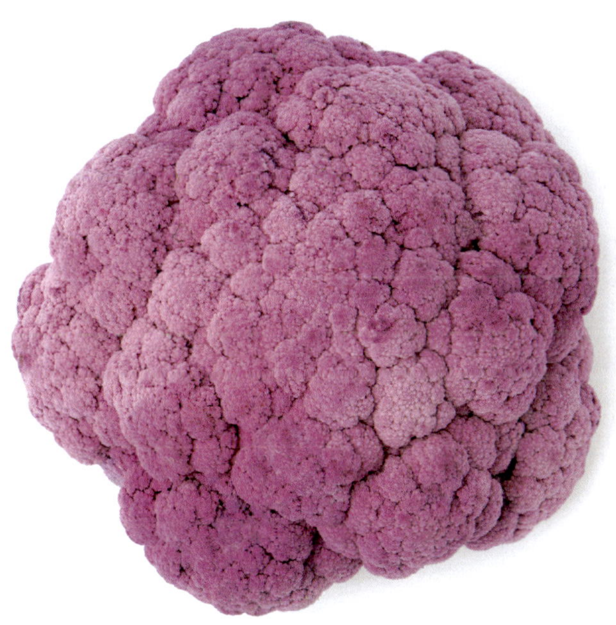

Purple Cauliflower.

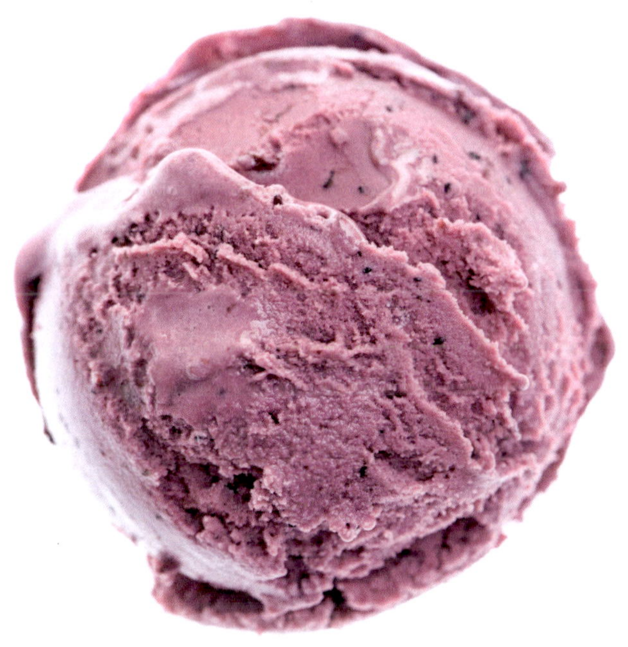

Cream, Skim Milk, Water, Sugar, Corn Syrup, Whey, Mono- and Diglycerides, Cellulose Gum, Guar Gum, Natural and Artificial Vanilla Flavor, Propylene Glycol, Pure Vanilla Extract, Natural and Artificial Flavors, Caramel Color, Salt, Polysorbate 80, Annatto, Turmeric, and Potassium Hydroxide.

FOOD

NOT FOOD

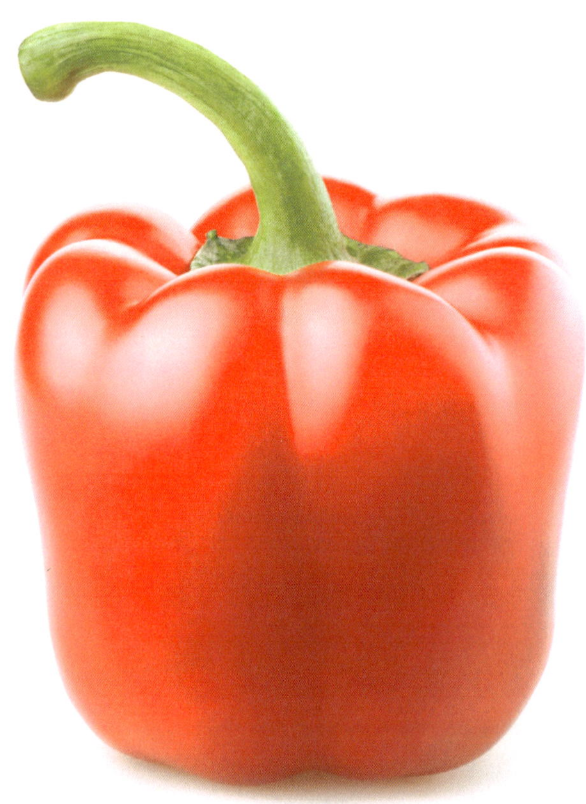

Red Bell Pepper.

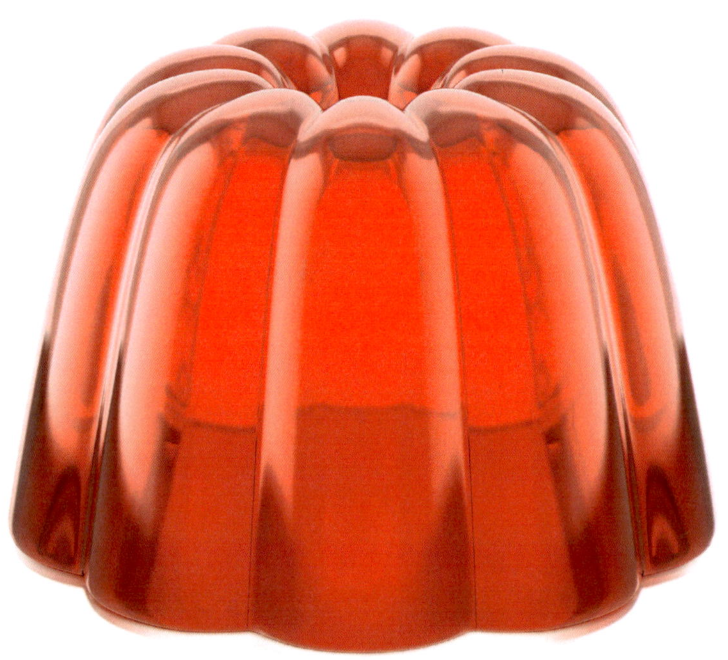

Sugar, Gelatin, Adipic Acid, Artificial Flavor, Disodium
Phosphate, Sodium Citrate, Fumaric Acid, Red #40,
and Blue #1.

FOOD

NOT FOOD

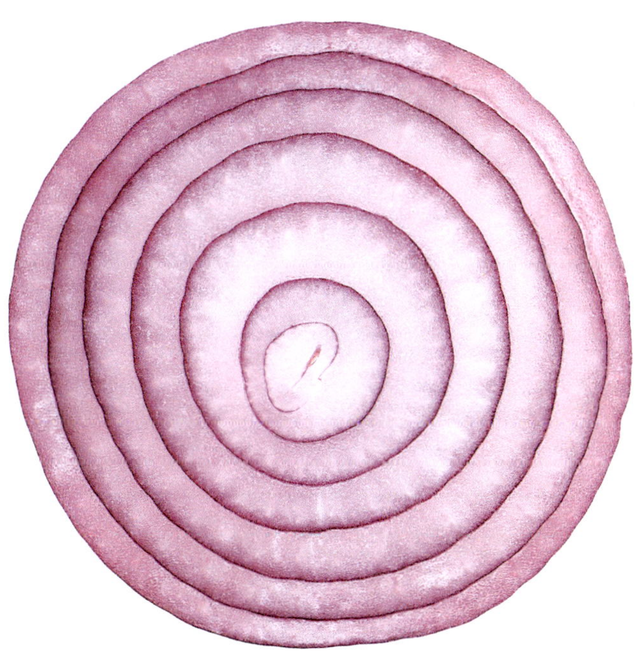

Red Onion.

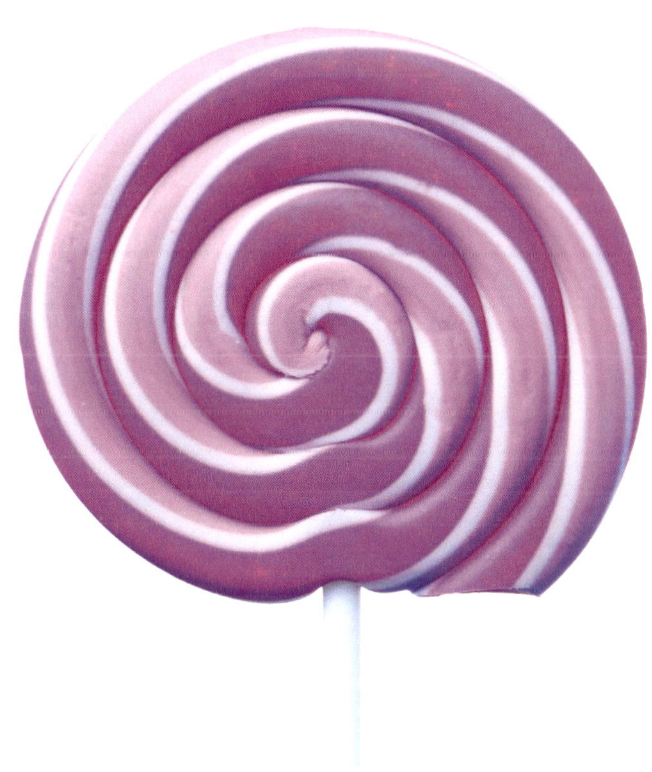

Sugar, Glucose Syrup, Water, Citric Acid, Artificial Flavors, Blue #1, Red #3, and Titanium Dioxide.

FOOD

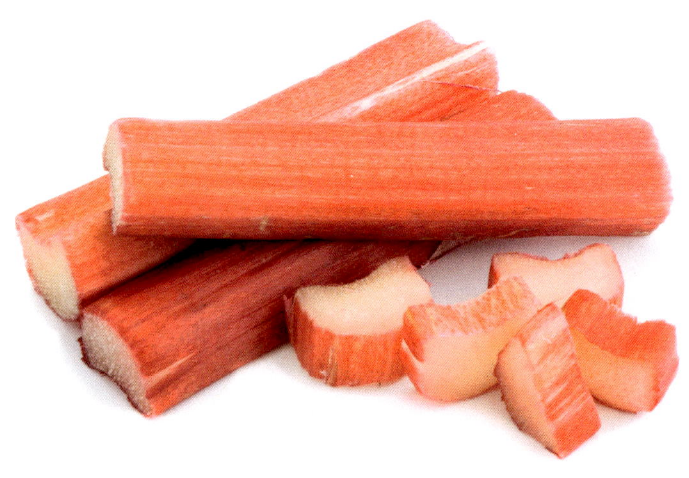

Rhubarb.

NOT FOOD

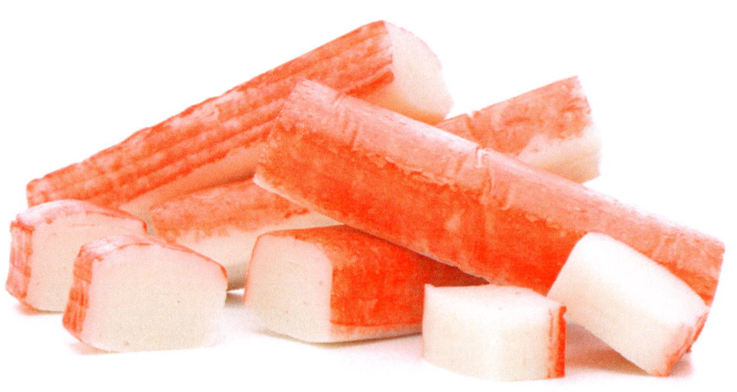

Alaska Pollock and/or Pacific Whiting, Water, Wheat Starch, Sugar, Egg Whites, Potato Starch, Sorbitol, Salt, Wheat Flour, Hydrolyzed Soy Protein, Crab Extract, Sodium Tripolyphosphate, Tetrasodium Pyrophosphate, Color Added, and Carmine Color.

FOOD

NOT FOOD

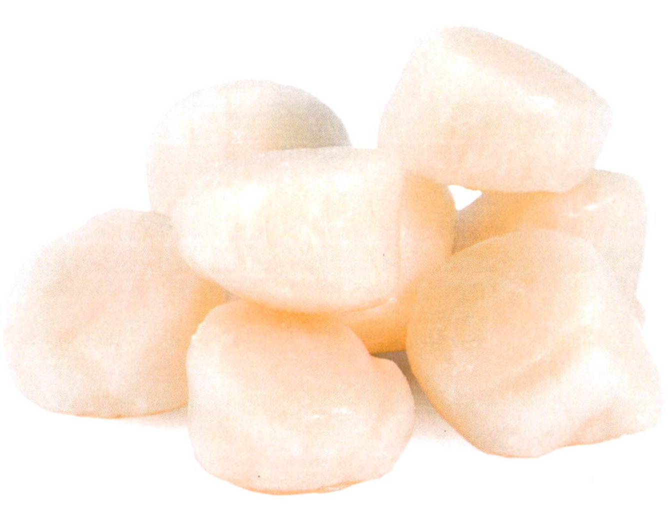

Scallops.

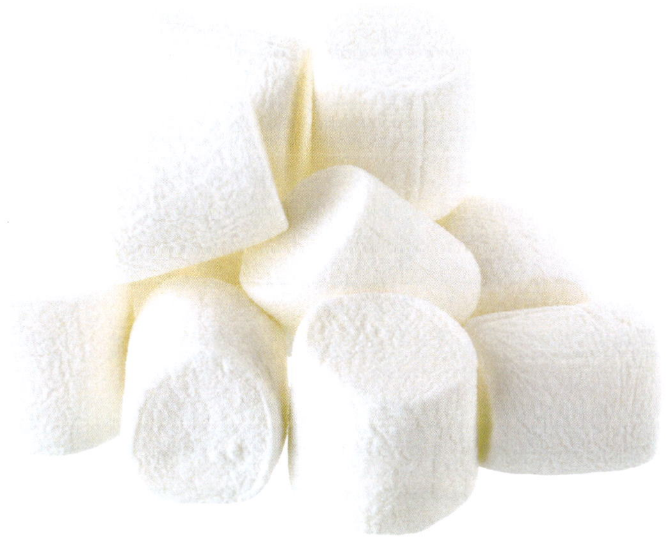

Corn Syrup, Sugar, Modified Cornstarch, Dextrose, Water, Gelatin, Tetrasodium Pyrophosphate, Natural and Artificial Flavor, and Blue #1.

FOOD

NOT FOOD

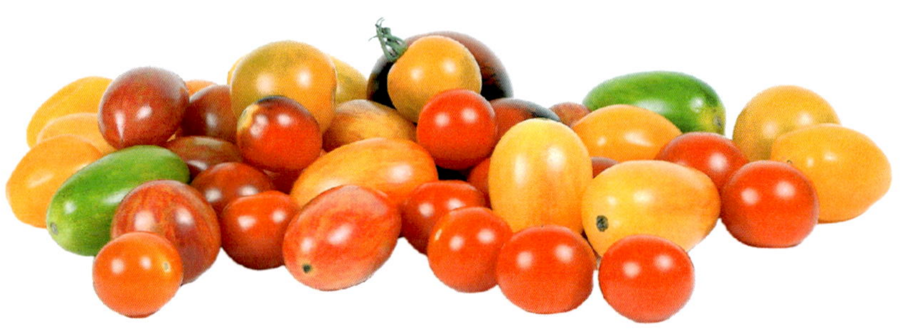

Tomatoes.

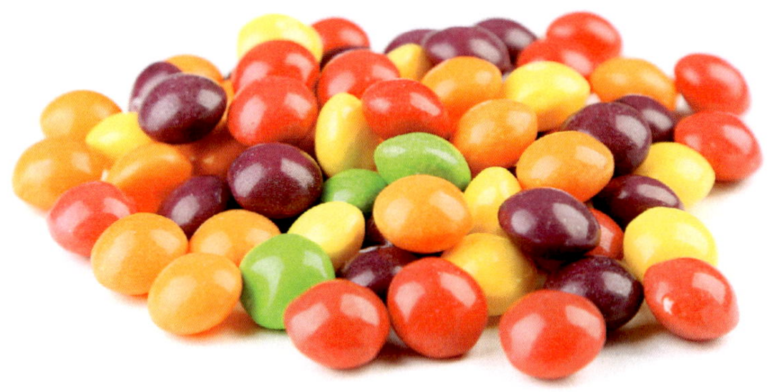

Sugar, Corn Syrup, Hydrogenated Palm Kernel Oil, Citric Acid, Tapioca Dextrin, Modified Corn Starch, Natural and Artificial Flavors, Red #40 Lake, Yellow #5 Lake, Blue #2 Lake, Yellow #6 Lake, Blue #1 Lake, Yellow #6, Red #40, Yellow #5, Blue #1, Titanium Dioxide, Sodium Citrate, and Carnauba Wax.

FOOD

NOT FOOD

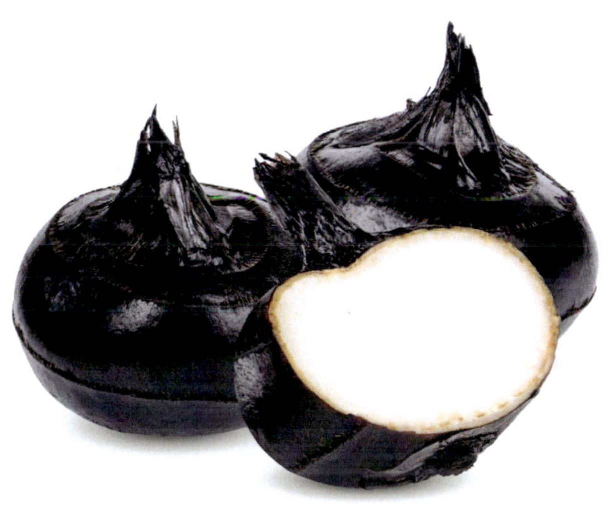

Water Chestnuts.

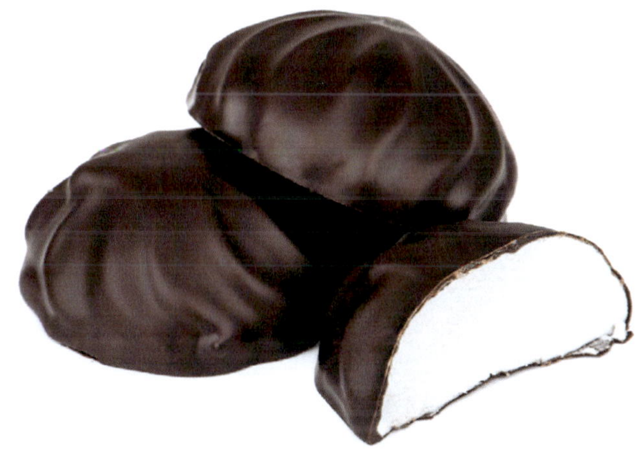

Glucose-Fructose Syrup, Sugar, Cocoa Mass, Cocoa Butter, Emulsifiers, Sunflower Lecithin, Natural Flavor, Wheat Flour, Vegetable Fat, Salt, Sodium Hydrogen Carbonate, Albumen, Sorbitol, and Agar-Agar.

FOOD

NOT FOOD

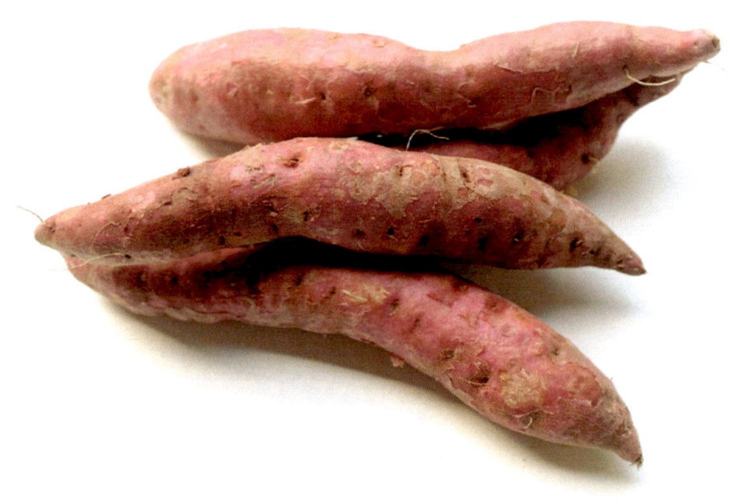

Yams.

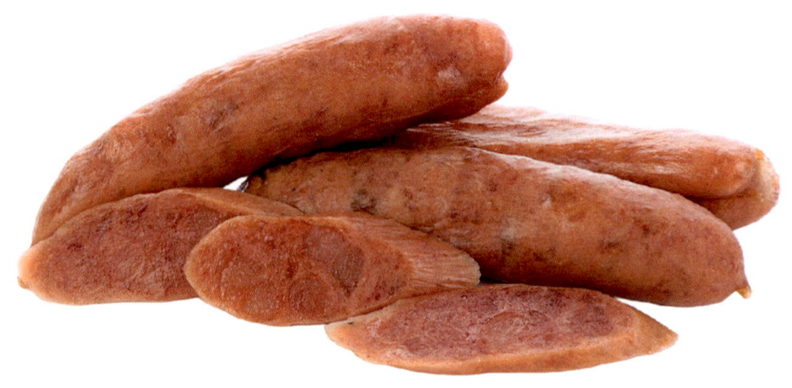

Beef, Pork, Water, Salt, Dextrose, Spices, Paprika, Lactic Acid Starter Culture, Sodium Erythorbate, Garlic Powder, Sodium Nitrite, Canola Oil, and Beef Collagen Casing.

FOOD

NOT FOOD

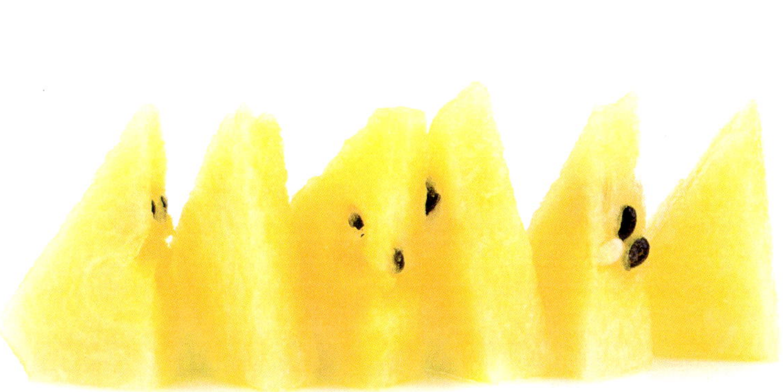

Yellow Watermelon.

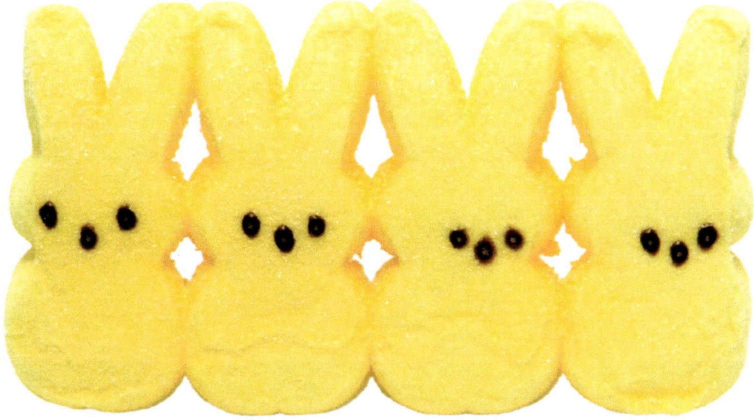

Sugar, Corn Syrup, Gelatin, Yellow #5, Potassium Sorbate, Natural Flavors, and Carnauba Wax.

FOOD

NOT FOOD

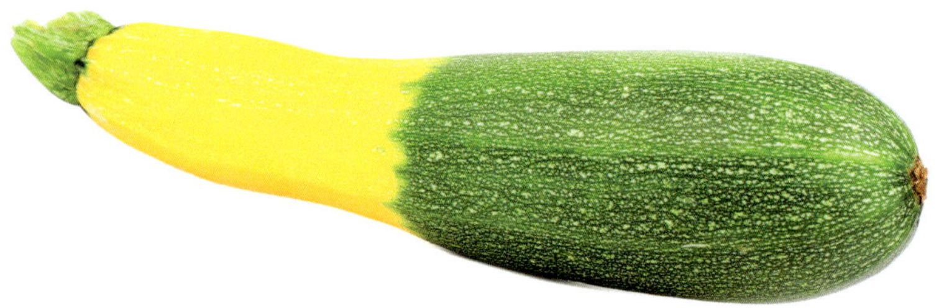

Zucchini.

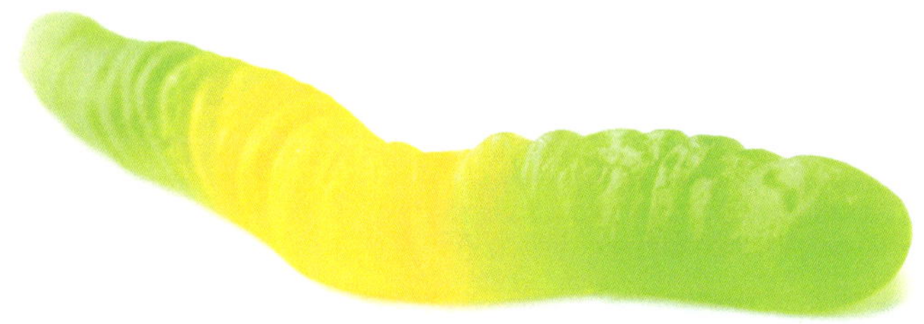

Corn Syrup, Sugar, Gelatin, Citric Acid, Pectin, Sorbitol, Natural and Artificial Flavors, Malic Acid, Carnauba Wax, Sodium Citrate, Yellow #6, Yellow #5, and Blue #1.

Hungry for more?

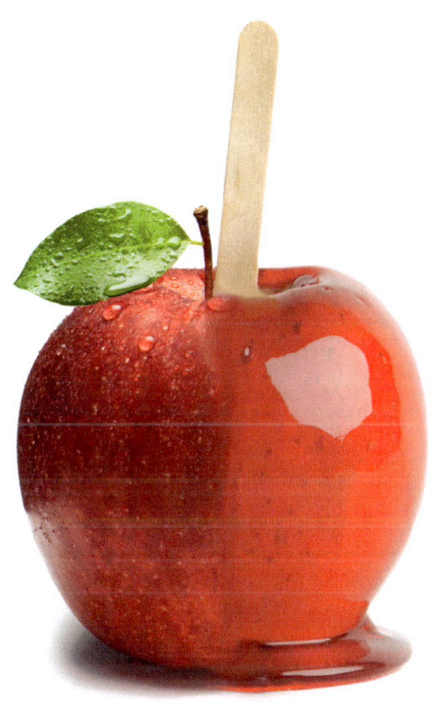

Visit
www.sweetpepperpublishing.com

ABOUT THE AUTHORS

Allison Bergman and Marcelle Sirkus are lifelong friends. Marcelle Sirkus is an award-winning screenwriter, creative producer, and musician. Allison Bergman is an accomplished stage and film director passionate about telling women's stories.

The authors' many collaborations include an award-winning comedy film, developing a television series — and co-producing a smash-hit playground cabaret show in the third grade.

Images and ingredients are for illustrative purposes only.
They do not represent any specific products or brands.